HowExpert Presents

How to Be an Equine Therapy Assistant

Your Step By Step Guide to Becoming a Therapeutic Horseback Riding Assistant

I0474875

HowExpert with Dana Feiwus

Copyright HowExpert™
www.HowExpert.com

For more tips related to this topic, visit HowExpert.com/equinetherapy.

Recommended Resources

- HowExpert.com – Quick 'How To' Guides on All Topics from A to Z by Everyday Experts.
- HowExpert.com/free – Free HowExpert Email Newsletter.
- HowExpert.com/books – HowExpert Books
- HowExpert.com/courses – HowExpert Courses
- HowExpert.com/clothing – HowExpert Clothing
- HowExpert.com/membership – HowExpert Membership Site
- HowExpert.com/affiliates – HowExpert Affiliate Program
- HowExpert.com/writers – Write About Your #1 Passion/Knowledge/Expertise & Become a HowExpert Author.
- HowExpert.com/resources – Additional HowExpert Recommended Resources
- YouTube.com/HowExpert – Subscribe to HowExpert YouTube.
- Instagram.com/HowExpert – Follow HowExpert on Instagram.
- Facebook.com/HowExpert – Follow HowExpert on Facebook.

Publisher's Foreword

Dear HowExpert reader,

HowExpert publishes quick 'how to' guides on all topics from A to Z by everyday experts.

At HowExpert, our mission is to discover, empower, and maximize talents of everyday people to ultimately make a positive impact in the world for all topics from A to Z...one everyday expert at a time!

All of our HowExpert guides are written by everyday people just like you and me who have a passion, knowledge, and expertise for a specific topic.

We take great pride in selecting everyday experts who have a passion, great writing skills, and knowledge about a topic that they love to be able to teach you about the topic you are also passionate about and eager to learn about.

We hope you get a lot of value from our HowExpert guides and it can make a positive impact in your life in some kind of way. All of our readers including you altogether help us continue living our mission of making a positive impact in the world for all spheres of influences from A to Z.

If you enjoyed one of our HowExpert guides, then please take a moment to send us your feedback from wherever you got this book.

Thank you and we wish you all the best in all aspects of life.

Sincerely,

BJ Min
Founder & Publisher of HowExpert
HowExpert.com

PS...If you are also interested in becoming a HowExpert author, then please visit our website at HowExpert.com/writers. Thank you & again, all the best!

Table of Contents

Introduction

Equine therapy, commonly called horse therapy, is growing popular among families searching for answers. Many children with a variety of physical and/or mental impairments qualify for this unique form of therapy. The therapy patients, referred to in this guide as riders, view horse therapy as a sport or a social activity rather than as therapy. Riding is not only fun—it has many benefits, most of which are visible immediately following lessons.

Benefits of Equine Therapy

Physical Benefits

- Riding gives patients a wider range of motion, specifically in the leg and torso muscles.
- The horse's pelvis forces the rider's pelvis to move correctly while in the saddle, effectively enabling the rider to walk better when out of the saddle.
- Riders gain muscle strength through a variety of exercises during lessons.
- Riders often vocalize louder and clearer while giving cues to the horses, which allows them to better articulate words off the horse as well.

Mental Benefits

- Controlling a 1,200-pound animal increases the rider's confidence.
- Riders receive praise during lessons, further boosting their confidence.
- The barn provides a safe haven where the riders can be themselves and make friends.
- Being in a positive environment teaches riders to embrace a positive attitude.
- Caring for the horses after lessons teaches the riders responsibility.

Social Benefits

- The community at a therapy barn (staff, volunteers, riders, and families) truly becomes a family unit, allowing riders to feel comfortable, safe, and loved.
- The riders create friendships with their fellow riders and volunteers.
- Weekly lessons give the riders something to look forward to and take pride in.
- Getting to know the riders and the therapy barn community provides a sense of "home" for the volunteers.

Who Does Equine Therapy Help?

Horse therapy is designed to benefit children and adults with any type of disability or impairment—for example, mental conditions like anxiety or autism. Horse therapy also benefits people suffering from physical impairments brought on by developmental problems, cerebral palsy, or accidental injuries.

Lessons are organized so that riders in each class are of similar age and capability. The instructor caters to the whole group at once, then works with individuals. Riders typically remain in the same class throughout the scheduled sessions, allowing them to bond with each other and their volunteers. This creates trust, which is essential, because the volunteers are responsible for the riders' safety.

The Importance of Family

It is vital to emphasize how important it is for the barn to be a warm and positive environment—a safe haven from the outside world. If the riders are comfortable and happy, they will focus on the instructor's directions and fully participate in lessons. Full participation is necessary for the riders to gain all the benefits offered by horse therapy.

Volunteers set the mood and environment of the barn, which contributes to the riders' success. It is important to greet the riders each week and get to know them. Riders look up to volunteers as mentors and friends. This relationship helps riders make the most out of each lesson.

Review

- Both adults and children with a variety of mental and physical impairments are eligible to participate in equine therapy.
- There are many mental, physical, and social benefits to riding that are noticeable immediately after lessons.
- The attitudes and actions of volunteers and staff members contribute to the environment at a therapy barn, which in turn contributes to the riders' experience there.

Chapter 1: How to Get Involved

Find a Barn Near You

When searching for a barn near you, start by searching on the internet for horse therapy barns in your area. Forums are also helpful. When you find a barn, read what people have to say about it and determine if it is a good fit for you.

The following link provides a list of many (but not all) equine therapy centers in the United States: **http://www.vetmed.ucdavis.edu/ccab/eatprog rams.htm**. Here, you can view therapy barns by state and city. Use this as a starting reference in your search.

Another great way to find a nearby therapy barn is through word of mouth. It is likely that someone you know is connected to a person eligible for horse therapy. Doctors may also know about local horse therapy barns if they recommend patients there. Utilize these sources when searching for a therapy barn.

Volunteer Training

Once you find a barn, the next step is to complete volunteer training. This must be done before you can participate in lessons. Training sessions are typically held before each session of lessons. You must fill out an information packet and attend a training session.

During training, the staff explains the program details and volunteer duties. You will meet the staff, and you will most likely watch an instructional video depicting what an actual lesson looks like. Then you will see the barn and arena where lessons take place. You should see a demonstration of how a horse is groomed and tacked (saddled), which must be done before each lesson.

After the tour and demonstrations, you can decide if you want to continue and sign up for lessons. Keep in mind that if you sign up for lessons, it is a commitment to be there every week for the duration of the session. If you cannot commit to a weekly time slot, horse therapy is not for you.

This commitment is necessary because the riders need a certain amount of volunteers to be able to ride. If volunteers don't show up, the riders cannot have their lesson, because it won't be safe for them. Go into horse therapy knowing that the time you volunteer is ongoing and essential to the riders' success. Also know that should you decide to volunteer, you will be immensely appreciated.

Volunteer Positions

Each barn has a unique set of volunteer positions available, but there are two that will always be necessary for carrying out lessons.

1. **Sidewalker**. It is the sidewalker's job to walk alongside the rider and horse. Many riders

need support to stay in the saddle; in that case, the rider has two sidewalkers: one on each side. The sidewalkers hold the riders' feet or legs, depending on how much support a particular rider needs, as they walk with the horse. They emphasize the instructor's directions, offer help with completing directions, and give praise when a rider follows the instructions and/or performs a technique well. If a rider does not need physical support to safely ride, often one sidewalker will accompany the rider, remaining at a close distance, to help with directions and give praise.

2. **Horse Leader**. While the sidewalker is in charge of the rider's safety, it is the horse leader's job to maintain control of the horse at all times. Excluding independent riders (who ride free of any volunteers), all other riders are given a horse leader. They control the horse with a lead rope attached to the bridle. This ensures that, even if the rider stops steering the horse, the lesson will not be disrupted; the horse leader can always redirect the horse to the desired position. If the rider is not yet capable of steering or stopping his or her horse, the horse leader takes full control during the lesson, while the sidewalkers teach the rider to use the reins and verbal cues. Barns have a variety of other volunteer positions, from bookkeepers to webmasters to snack providers. Each position is important for keeping morale high, which allows everyone to focus on the mission of therapeutic riding.

Horse Leader Training

Immediately following a volunteer training session, you are qualified to be a sidewalker. For those who wish to be a horse leader, certain prerequisites are required. For instance, you must have a certain amount of experience around horses. Anyone who has owned a horse or has been professionally trained to ride is qualified. However, those individuals must still go through horse leader training.

Horse leader training is held to ensure that everyone in the barn handles the horses in the same manner. Many people walk through the barn every day, but it is best if staff and volunteers handle the horses uniformly. A routine helps the horses feel at ease around so many strangers.

The new horse leaders are taught how their particular barn wishes to handle the horses. They are also taught the mounting processes. A therapy rider mounts a horse differently than an able-bodied rider. Often times, the mounting process is stressful to the horses, so the horse leaders must control the horses and make them comfortable during mounting.

Once the new horse leaders are trained, they are free to sign up for lessons and be fully responsible for the horses.

Review

- Once you find a barn near you, volunteer training sessions will provide the necessary information to teach lessons and enhance the riders' experience.
- There are two main volunteer positions in equine therapy: the sidewalker (who assists the rider) and the horse leader (who controls the horse).
- Horse leaders receive more training than sidewalkers and generally have more barn experience, so they make great mentors for volunteers who need help adjusting.

Chapter 2: How a Therapy Barn Differs From a Normal Barn

Tack

A lot of the tack (such as saddles, blankets, and stirrups) used at a therapy barn is the same used at other barns. However, there are differences in some items. There is also additional equipment to make riding easier and help the riders achieve the correct body positions.

Tack varies from barn to barn, but the most common therapy riding tack is:

<u>Sidepull</u>

A sidepull is very similar to a bridle. It fits and looks similarly. But a sidepull doesn't have a bit, which is the metal bar that rests inside the horse's mouth. In a therapy session, many riders yank on the reins, sometimes uncontrollably, and it could be harmful and irritating to the horse if a bit was used. Instead, the sidepull has a band that wraps around the horse's muzzle. The pressure on the horse's face caused by tugging the reins tells the horse which way to turn.

Reins

A variety of reins are used in therapy riding. These are the most common two.

- **Rainbow reins**. The most common reins are called rainbow reins. They are marked with different colors up and down the leather, making it easy for a sidewalker to tell the rider where to hold them. For example, if a rider is holding the reins too loosely, the sidewalker can say, "Hold the reins on the red," and the rider will know the proper place for their hands.
- **Handle reins**. These reins are made of nylon and have two handles for the riders to grip. When holding the handles correctly, it looks like the rider is on a bicycle. These reins are easier for riders to grip during a lesson.

Risers

A riser is a piece of foam shaped to fit under the saddle. It is thicker in the back, causing the seat-portion of the saddle to rise. This is used for riders who need help sitting straight and tall in their saddle. The lift forces their body to straighten, which exercises the rider's core muscles.

Some tack remains unaltered: the saddle, the girth (which holds the saddle around the horse like a belt), the stirrups and stirrup leathers (which connect the stirrups to the saddle), and the blanket (which goes under the saddle for comfort).

Most therapy riders use English tack as opposed to Western tack. Riding with English tack incorporates more muscle movement. There are many differences between English and Western tack. First, the Western saddle is bigger and heavier than the English saddle. The girth (commonly called a cinch with Western tack) and stirrups are connected to the saddle. There's also a saddle horn, which cowboys used for lassoing. The English saddle is significantly smaller and lighter. Everything breaks down into various pieces (saddle, girth, stirrup leathers, and stirrups). The rider can feel more of the horse's movements through the English saddle since it is smaller, increasing the benefits of riding.

Horse Temperaments

It takes a particular type of horse to be a "therapist." Many donated horses do not qualify to serve in therapy sessions.

A good therapy horse must have the following characteristics of temperament:

Quiet

Horses spook easily by nature. Something as small as a gust of wind can send a horse running. A quiet horse does not spook as easily as others. This is important for many reasons. For example, if a child riding a horse decides to scream, most horses would spook and run, but a quiet horse would not.

Gentle

A therapy horse must be gentle for the safety of riders and volunteers. Many volunteers are not familiar with horse behavior. For instance, mares (female horses) do not like their hindquarters touched or leaned on. If a volunteer does not know this and starts vigorously brushing a mare's hindquarters, the horse could get angry and kick. However, a gentle mare would have a smaller, less dangerous reaction and settle down soon after.

Trained Well

A therapy horse must respond well to verbal and physical cues. If a rider gives a cue, such as pulling the reins back to stop, the horse must comply. If not, the rider will start to pull harder and harder until the horse gets angry. A well-trained horse knows the routine of lessons and soothes the rider and volunteers.

Therapy horses are the kindest horses. They work hard and resist many aspects of natural horse behavior. It is important to praise the horses, as well as the riders, for their behavior and respectfulness.

Even the best horses have moody or irritable moments. In those cases, let them rest until they regain their composure. The horses are the most essential part of equine therapy, and they truly become part of the barn family.

A Relaxing Yet Structured Environment

A therapy barn is a peaceful place—an escape from the harshness of everyday life. It is a place where riders feel accepted and appreciated for who they are, something they may not regularly experience. In order to maintain that feeling of unquestionable comfort, everyone needs to feel safe and protected.

There are safety rules regarding mounting and conduct during lessons, and there are safety rules regarding bad weather and emergencies. Volunteers must be aware of the safety rules set by their barn. Rain, lightening, tornadoes, and fires are all reasons to promptly end a lesson and get the riders and horses to safety.

Review

- Much of the tack used at a therapy barn is unique. Consult an instructor if you come across an unfamiliar piece of equipment so it can be used properly.
- Therapy horses are the world's mellowest horses. Respect them and develop a relationship to reduce the potential for injury and improve the quality of therapy sessions.
- Though the barn is a peaceful place, certain safety rules must be followed.

Chapter 3: How to Handle the Horses

Catching

It is the horse leader's job to retrieve the horse before each lesson. This may entail bringing a horse in from its stall in the barn or "catching" a horse out in the pasture. Because the horse leaders have more training, barns typically only allow them to enter horse pastures.

Catching is demonstrated during training. It involves bringing a halter (a head harness) and a lead rope into the pasture and finding the horse you need for the lesson. Once you find the correct horse, sling the lead rope over its neck to keep it from walking away. Fit the halter over its face. Then you buckle the harness, gather up the lead rope, and walk the horse out to the saddle bay (the area where you tack horses).

General Handling

All volunteers are given advice and protocol on how to handle horses. Therapy barns should handle horses consistently so they develop routines and adjust better to strangers.

Here are some best practices for handling a horse:

- Go around the horse by circling around the front, rather than the back, of its body. If you do go around the back, be sure to let the horse know by placing your hand softly on the horse's side and dragging it with you around the horse. If a horse hears noise behind it, it might kick; but if it knows a person is back there, it will stay calm.
- Always be aware of horses' ears. Horses display their moods with their ears. If a horse has its ears pinned back, it is angry or irritated. This is frequently accompanied by flaring nostrils and stomping. In that case, step back and let the horse calm down. However, there is a difference between pinned ears and ears that are simply turned to hear what is happening behind them. Horses are curious and will listen to noises in all directions. This is nothing to worry about.
- Horses cannot see directly in front of them. Rather, they see from the sides. Never approach a horse from the front unless you're speaking and the horse can hear you coming. Instead, approach from the side. Horses spook easily, and it is their instinct to kick or run when get scared. Keeping the horse at ease helps both the horse's behavioral stability and the person's safety.
- If you ever need to give a physical cue to a horse, such as pushing it to the side a few steps, be sure to release the pressure immediately following the horse's compliance. Horses naturally move away from pressure, so if you push on a horse's left side, it will step to the right. However, if you keep applying pressure,

the horse will continue to move away from it while growing angry. The reward for a horse complying with your command is to simply stop applying that command. They also appreciate a good massage!

- When feeding a horse by hand (for example, giving a carrot as a reward after a lesson), be sure to keep your hand flat and your fingers together. If your fingers are separated or bent, the horse may bite them.

- It is against the rules to let riders feed horses by hand. Instead, have the rider place food items in a bucket and offer them to the horse. Insert carrots into sections of hollow pool noodles for safe "carrot feeders."

Grooming and Tacking

Volunteers are asked to arrive 45 minutes before each lesson to groom and tack the horses in preparation for the riders' arrival. Obviously, tacking is necessary, but you may be wondering why it is important to groom too. Grooming ensures the comfort and cleanliness of the horses. If mud is matted into their hair and you put a saddle on top of that, it will rub against their skin and cause sores or rashes. Similarly, their hooves must be clean, because a small rock lodged into the bottom can also cause discomfort and poor behavior during a lesson.

Here is a list of commonly-used grooming tools:

Curry Comb

This comb is often round or oval and is covered in blunted protrusions. It is designed to raise dirt and loose hair from the undercoat to the surface of the horse's hair when rubbed in circular motions. This is the first of three brushes used to clean a horse's hair.

Hard Brush

The hard brush has long, thick bristles. It is designed to wipe away dirt and loose hair released by the curry comb. The proper way to use it is to sweep it with the nap of the hair (from the horse's front to its back) and flick your wrist at the end of each stroke. This ensures that dirt is swept off the horse's body.

Soft Brush

The soft brush has soft, fine bristles. It removes anything the hard brush missed. It is also used in more sensitive areas, such as the face and neck.

Hoof Pick

The hoof pick is a tool for cleaning the hooves. It has a handle and a two-sided top, like an axe. One side has a blunted pick and the other has a brush with short, firm bristles. The pick is used to scrape mud, rocks, and other nuisances out of the crevice underneath the horse's foot. The brush is used to remove mud from the outside of the hoof. All volunteers are taught how to properly lift a horse's leg in order to clean the hooves.

Hairbrush

A common human hairbrush may be used to brush out the mane and tail if muddy or matted, or simply for appearance's sake.

After a horse is fully groomed, it is ready to be tacked, which means putting the tack on the horse. Grooming and tacking is a joint effort between the sidewalkers and horse leaders. With two or more people working on each horse, the job gets done quickly. The remaining time can be used to prepare further, such as setting up trail patterns in the arena, or relax before the lesson begins.

Here is a list of the essential tack:

Blanket

The blanket is laid across the horse's back first. It protects the horse from being rubbed by the saddle.

Saddle

The saddle is placed directly on top of the blanket.
With most riders, English saddles are used because
they promote use of core muscles.

Girth

The girth is the "belt" that straps the saddle to the
horse's body. It buckles onto the saddle on both sides
and can be loosened or tightened. Often, a horse will
suck in air as the girth is being attached and then
release the air later, so the girth will need to be
tightened.

Stirrups

The stirrups are separate from the saddle when using
English tack. In order to attach them, you must slide
stirrup leathers through the holes on top of the
stirrups. The stirrup leathers can then be buckled onto
the saddle.

Sidepull

The sidepull is the equivalent of the bridle for therapy
riding, but without a bit. This is strapped over the
horse's face and a lead rope is connected under the
chin for the horse leader's use.

Reins

Reins are attached to the sidepull. They allow the rider to control the horse. Pulling side to side tells the horse to turn, while pulling back tells the horse to stop. A squeeze of the legs and the verbal cue "walk on" tells the horse to go.

Other specialty tack may be used for some riders. Please see the section "Tack" under the topic "How a Therapy Barn Differs From A Normal Barn."

Respect the Horses During Lessons

The rule "treat others as you'd like to be treated" applies to any barn setting. Horses are big, heavy, and strong animals. They can be dangerous under the wrong circumstances. But if you handle them correctly and respect their space, they are a pleasure to work with. Horses will give back what they get.

If you act according to the tips given here and spend time getting to know a horse's personality, that horse will begin to remember you and consider you a "friend." Horses are very peaceful and loving, and as long as you show that corresponding side of yourself to them, a mutual respect for each other will be developed and strengthened.

Review

- After the horse leader catches the horse, he or she and the sidewalkers work together to groom and tack the horse for the lesson
- Be aware of the horse you are working with to ensure it remains content. An angry horse is a dangerous horse.
- Treat the horses as though they are part of the team, because they are. In fact, they are the most important part.

Chapter 4: Riders

Praise, Help, Support

Many of the benefits of therapy riding relate to improving confidence. It is up to the volunteers and instructors to offer ample praise when a rider performs a task or technique well. Praise is always given when a rider tries something. The abilities of riders vary widely, so sometimes a rider gets praise because he or she has performed a technique perfectly, and sometimes a rider receives praise simply for holding the reins in the correct position. The idea is to get riders to do a little more than they did they week before. The goal of therapy riding is to steer the riders toward being able to ride independently.

It is up to the sidewalkers to offer help if the rider asks for it or is clearly struggling. If a rider is having trouble holding the reins correctly, the sidewalker can physically take his or her hands and put them on the correct spot. Sometimes, when a rider is shown that way, they remember it for next time.

The most important aspect of helping riders during lessons is to provide the correct level of support. For example, some riders can sit on their horses with no problems, while others need support to remain safely in the saddle.

There are several holds a sidewalker can use to ensure the safety of the rider:

Cuff Hold

This is when a sidewalker holds onto the cuff of the rider's pants. This provides indirect support. It gives the sidewalker contact with the rider in case something should go wrong.

Ankle Hold

This is when a sidewalker holds the ankle or heel of the rider. In this case, there will most likely be a sidewalker on either side of the rider, both holding an ankle or heel. This is used when a rider is comfortable sitting in their saddle, but needs extra support while trotting or help if they start to slide from the center.

Thigh Hold

This is when a sidewalker uses the arm nearest to the horse to grab the front of the saddle and lay the forearm across the rider's thigh. This is used when a rider cannot stay in the center of his or her saddle alone. It is a physical and tiring hold, so it is common of sidewalkers to switch sides during lessons to rest their muscles.

Special Cases

There are some special cases where absolute, full-sidewalker support is necessary. For example, if a rider has no means of controlling his or her body, the sidewalker will need to hold that rider's torso in an erect position. In these special cases, the instructor will help the sidewalkers find a comfortable way to keep the rider safe.

Be a Mentor and a Friend

Apart from keeping the riders safe, the volunteers are there to keep them happy. Riders often view therapy riding not as another form of therapy, but as a sport or a social activity, something that they do not normally get to participate in. They get excited to see their "helpers" and their horses. The barn is a place for them to let down their guard and be themselves. The more interaction there is between riders and volunteers, the more the riders' confidence grows.

A friendship with a rider benefits the volunteers as well. Being a part of such an immense change in someone's life creates a powerful bond between rider and volunteer. There is mutual trust and respect, and for volunteers, a strong sense of pride in the riders' accomplishments. The people at a therapy barn truly become a second family to the riders.

Review

- A combination of ample praise and repetition of instructions helps the rider to achieve a higher skill level and understanding.
- Using the proper supportive hold, as specified by the instructor, ensures that the rider is safe in his or her saddle.
- Befriending riders is beneficial to staff members and volunteers.

Chapter 5: Lessons

Mounting

Mounting at a therapy barn is a different process. It takes special equipment and several people to perform the task correctly and safely. There are two ways to mount, depending on the rider's needs: the block and the ramp.

Mounting Block

This is simply a platform with steps leading up to it. Before the rider approaches the block, the horse must be led to it. To do this, first a sidewalker stands parallel and about two feet away from the block, creating a "human wall" for the horse to stand inside. Then the horse leader brings the horse in between the block and the sidewalker. The rider is then directed up the steps and the instructor lifts the rider into the saddle. Once mounted, the group walks out of the block, a second sidewalker can then join if necessary, and the stirrups are adjusted to fit the rider correctly. The lesson begins once all riders are mounted.

Mounting Ramp

This consists of two parallel ramps that are significantly taller than the block. It's used for riders that are too big to lift up into the saddle. A sidewalker walks up one side of the ramp while the instructor helps the rider up the other side. The horse is then led in between the two ramps and the instructor and sidewalker help the rider into the saddle.

Warm Ups, Trail Patterns, Trotting, Two Point, Techniques, and Games

Each lesson starts with warm ups. The riders take laps around the arena while everyone is mounted. There are one to four riders per lesson. Then the exercises begin. These are a variety of stretches designed to engage the rider's whole body. The rider is instructed to drop their reins and let their horse leader take full control while the exercises are performed.

Here is a list of examples of stretches or exercises:

- Torso Twists
- Stretching arms forward to the horse's ears and backward to the horse's tail
- Reaching the arms up, out, and down to their own toes
- Steering exercises to sync the rider with their horse

After warmups, the lesson can go in a variety of directions. A common activity is to go through an obstacle course-like arrangement called a trail pattern, which can be set up differently each lesson.

This helps the riders by practicing learned techniques and incorporating intellectual activities with physical activities.

Some aspects of the trail pattern:

- Walking over ground poles (wooden poles set up in the arena)
- Weaving around cones or poles
- Steering through a short maze
- Turning in tight right angles, as opposed to more gradual circular turns
- Walking in figure eights or other patterns

Trotting is a favorite for many riders. Humans have three gaits: walk, jog, and run. Horses have four gaits: walk, trot, cantor, and gallop. Riders remain at the walk and trot levels until they begin riding independently and can safely cantor. The trot reinforces many skills learned by the riders, such as holding their heads straight up, using reins to steer, and hugging the horse with their legs.

The trot also gives riders the opportunity to learn a new technique called posting. Posting is the when the rider uses his or her legs to move up and down in the saddle along with the horse's motions; this strengthens the leg muscles and is easier on the horse's back, since the rider is no longer slamming down on the horse with each step. Posting at a trot engages the rider completely (physically and mentally), proving a useful tool for the rider's success.

Two-point is a technique commonly used among able-bodied riders. To perform this technique, which is more like a position, the rider reaches forward to the horse's mane, leans his or her shoulders into the reach, and lifts his or her bottom out of the saddle with the knees remaining bent. It looks almost like the rider is leaning down to hug the horse's neck. This position is used by the rider when a horse is jumping. The purpose is to protect the horse's spine from receiving too much pressure. Therapy riders do not jump (unless they are highly advanced), but the two-point position is used in nearly every lesson because it works the leg muscles and forces the rider to concentrate harder. In most cases, it is incorporated into the trail patterns; for example, the riders are asked to two-point while they walk over the ground poles. However the position is utilized, the riders are receiving the benefits of physical exertion and mental stimulation.

Various techniques are taught over the course of a session, interspersed among lessons. Here is a list of some techniques:

- Holding the reins and steering properly
- Cues to the horse, verbal and physical (for example, tapping the feet into the horse's belly tells the horse to walk)
- Positioning the body to sit straight and tall
- Look in the direction the rider intends to go
- The recognition of parts of the horse and other general horse knowledge

Many lessons, mostly those with young children, end with some sort of game. These fun activities incorporate riding skills and horse knowledge.

Here is a list of some fun game ideas for equine therapy lessons:

- Musical Horses (like musical chairs): teaches steering, walking, and stopping
- Red Light, Green Light: teaches walking and stopping
- Missing Animals (scattered stuffed animals are retrieved and returned to the instructor): teaches steering with intent
- Trivia Games (the rider answers questions about horses and/or riding in order to move toward the finish line): stimulates intellect
- Relay Race (riders carry an object to a barrel or bucket on the other side of the arena then come back to tag in the next rider): teaches teamwork and steering with intent

Dismounting

At the end of each lesson, the horse leaders line up the horses in the arena and the instructor dismounts all the riders. There are several methods used to dismount riders, but dismounting is always the responsibility of the instructor. The sidewalkers may assist in the dismount by helping a rider swing his or her legs over the horse. The horse leader maintains control over the horse during this process. Once on the ground, the rider can hold the end of the horse's lead rope and help lead the horse back to the saddle bay for untacking.

Untacking, Grooming, and Feeding with Riders

If the riders are able and willing, they are encouraged to untack their horses. This is the process of removing the saddle and equipment and putting it away in the tack room. The riders are also encouraged to brush their horses and interact with them on the ground. This develops their sense of responsibility and confidence.

Horses love eating treats just as much as humans do, and some of their favorite treats are carrots. If riders bring carrots, they can offer them to their horses as a reward after untacking. However, riders must use a designated "carrot feeder" while feeding so their fingers are not accidentally bitten.

The rider finishes and says goodbye to everyone, horse and human. The horse leader then delivers the horse to its proper place, whether that be a stall in the barn or into pasture.

Review

- There are two ways to mount riders: the mounting block and the mounting ramp.
- Each lesson consists of a variety of warm-up stretches, exercises, and games that strengthen riders and engage their whole body and mind.

- After dismounting, the riders are encouraged to help untack, groom, and feed their horses to learn responsibility and social interaction.

Chapter 6: Aftermath

Physical and Mental Changes Within Riders

Visible changes can be seen from week to week as riders participate in lessons. I have personally witnessed much improvement in all the riders I have worked with. These improvements give the riders a strong sense of accomplishment. They gain pride with each achievement, no matter the size. Volunteers are just as proud as the riders' families. Below is a list of a few of the improvements I've observed among riders in horse therapy:

- Riders with cerebral palsy can walk more naturally after dismounting
    - Bigger, longer steps
    - Straightened legs
    - More stability
    - Less support needed
- Riders with communication impairments talk and use physical cues
    - "Walk on" to make the horse go
    - Often learn to say their horse's name
    - Singing along with music during lessons
- Riders with physical ailments gain strength
    - Legs grow stronger, allows the rider to stabilize themselves in the saddle
    - Riders begin to help carry tack back to the barn
    - Riders need less support while on and off the horse

- Riders with attention-deficit or learning disabilities gain focus
  - Riders become engaged in the lesson activities
  - Riders learn to follow directions
  - Less reliance on the sidewalkers for instruction reminders
  - Less distractions from events outside the arena as the riders become absorbed with the lesson activities
- Riders in wheelchairs begin to walk
  - Body adjusts to movement patterns of the horse and mimics them
  - Riders gain muscle strength for further support
- Riders gain confidence
  - Riders perform techniques without hesitation
  - Riders gain comfort around large animals and unfamiliar people
  - Riders get excited each week to do something they excel in

Being a Part of Something Bigger Than Yourself

One of my fellow volunteers once said that with most volunteer gigs, you give a few hours or a day or maybe a week, but with therapy riding you give a piece of yourself. What a wonderful way to describe it! If you decide to volunteer—if you decide that you really want to give back—I cannot think of a better way to dramatically improve the lives of others that are often ignored and even mistreated. The joy that envelops a therapy barn is infectious and will flow out into your everyday life. I am proud to say, without hesitation, that my second home is a barn, and no, the smell does not bother me.

More Volunteer Opportunities

For those who do not particularly want to work with horses, there are other volunteer opportunities available at therapy barns. It takes a lot of people to run the program efficiently and every bit of help drives a barn closer to its mission.

Here is a list of some of other positions and duties that aid a therapy barn:

Webmaster

A barn's website is a great way to communicate with volunteers. An up-to-date website makes communication easier.

Bookkeeper

Since therapy barns are nonprofit organizations, it is important to keep track of finance and use funds diligently.

Fundraising

Barns must raise money to improve programs and keep horses in shape.

Snacks

For large gatherings where volunteers are needed, snacks and meals are offered in appreciation of their time and devotion.

Mail

From stuffing envelopes to sending emails, a barn must communicate with volunteers, donors, riders, and potential patrons.

Review

- Visible and audible effects of riding are seen each week as the riders gain strength and courage, among other accumulated traits.
- Being in the center of such inspiring life improvements provides volunteers with a sense of pride and belonging.
- If this sounds interesting to you, but you are not a horse person, do not be discouraged—

there are other opportunities for volunteer
work at all therapy barns!

About the Expert

My name is Dana Feiwus. I am a recent graduate of the University of North Texas with a major in English, Creative Writing. I began volunteering at ManeGait Therapeutic Horsemanship in McKinney, Texas two years ago because I was always fond of horses. However, I soon learned that therapy riding is about much more than horses, and I have been there almost every weekend since I began. From weekly lessons to fundraising events to the annual horse show, there is no place I would rather spend my free time.

Though I have worked with many riders, one rider in particular holds a special place in my heart. This five-year-old girl with cerebral palsy and I shared our first lesson at ManeGait together and two years later she's now walking with no support and riding like a champ. As much as riding has improved her life, she has undoubtedly improved mine as well.

HowExpert publishes quick 'how to' guides on all topics from A to Z by everyday experts. Visit HowExpert.com to learn more.

Recommended Resources

- HowExpert.com – Quick 'How To' Guides on All Topics from A to Z by Everyday Experts.
- HowExpert.com/free – Free HowExpert Email Newsletter.
- HowExpert.com/books – HowExpert Books
- HowExpert.com/courses – HowExpert Courses
- HowExpert.com/clothing – HowExpert Clothing
- HowExpert.com/membership – HowExpert Membership Site
- HowExpert.com/affiliates – HowExpert Affiliate Program
- HowExpert.com/writers – Write About Your #1 Passion/Knowledge/Expertise & Become a HowExpert Author.
- HowExpert.com/resources – Additional HowExpert Recommended Resources
- YouTube.com/HowExpert – Subscribe to HowExpert YouTube.
- Instagram.com/HowExpert – Follow HowExpert on Instagram.
- Facebook.com/HowExpert – Follow HowExpert on Facebook.